The charter of the Royal Canal Company, with their rules, and extracts from the act of the 29th of His present Majesty George III. With an index. To which is prefixed, a list of the subscribers.

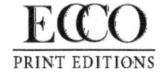

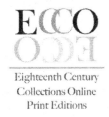

Eighteenth Century
Collections Online
Print Editions

Gale ECCO Print Editions

Relive history with *Eighteenth Century Collections Online*, now available in print for the independent historian and collector. This series includes the most significant English-language and foreign-language works printed in Great Britain during the eighteenth century, and is organized in seven different subject areas including literature and language; medicine, science, and technology; and religion and philosophy. The collection also includes thousands of important works from the Americas.

The eighteenth century has been called "The Age of Enlightenment." It was a period of rapid advance in print culture and publishing, in world exploration, and in the rapid growth of science and technology – all of which had a profound impact on the political and cultural landscape. At the end of the century the American Revolution, French Revolution and Industrial Revolution, perhaps three of the most significant events in modern history, set in motion developments that eventually dominated world political, economic, and social life.

In a groundbreaking effort, Gale initiated a revolution of its own: digitization of epic proportions to preserve these invaluable works in the largest online archive of its kind. Contributions from major world libraries constitute over 175,000 original printed works. Scanned images of the actual pages, rather than transcriptions, recreate the works *as they first appeared.*

Now for the first time, these high-quality digital scans of original works are available via print-on-demand, making them readily accessible to libraries, students, independent scholars, and readers of all ages.

For our initial release we have created seven robust collections to form one the world's most comprehensive catalogs of 18th century works.

Initial Gale ECCO Print Editions collections include:

History and Geography
Rich in titles on English life and social history, this collection spans the world as it was known to eighteenth-century historians and explorers. Titles include a wealth of travel accounts and diaries, histories of nations from throughout the world, and maps and charts of a world that was still being discovered. Students of the War of American Independence will find fascinating accounts from the British side of conflict.

Social Science

Delve into what it was like to live during the eighteenth century by reading the first-hand accounts of everyday people, including city dwellers and farmers, businessmen and bankers, artisans and merchants, artists and their patrons, politicians and their constituents. Original texts make the American, French, and Industrial revolutions vividly contemporary.

Medicine, Science and Technology

Medical theory and practice of the 1700s developed rapidly, as is evidenced by the extensive collection, which includes descriptions of diseases, their conditions, and treatments. Books on science and technology, agriculture, military technology, natural philosophy, even cookbooks, are all contained here.

Literature and Language

Western literary study flows out of eighteenth-century works by Alexander Pope, Daniel Defoe, Henry Fielding, Frances Burney, Denis Diderot, Johann Gottfried Herder, Johann Wolfgang von Goethe, and others. Experience the birth of the modern novel, or compare the development of language using dictionaries and grammar discourses.

Religion and Philosophy

The Age of Enlightenment profoundly enriched religious and philosophical understanding and continues to influence present-day thinking. Works collected here include masterpieces by David Hume, Immanuel Kant, and Jean-Jacques Rousseau, as well as religious sermons and moral debates on the issues of the day, such as the slave trade. The Age of Reason saw conflict between Protestantism and Catholicism transformed into one between faith and logic -- a debate that continues in the twenty-first century.

Law and Reference

This collection reveals the history of English common law and Empire law in a vastly changing world of British expansion. Dominating the legal field is the *Commentaries of the Law of England* by Sir William Blackstone, which first appeared in 1765. Reference works such as almanacs and catalogues continue to educate us by revealing the day-to-day workings of society.

Fine Arts

The eighteenth-century fascination with Greek and Roman antiquity followed the systematic excavation of the ruins at Pompeii and Herculaneum in southern Italy; and after 1750 a neoclassical style dominated all artistic fields. The titles here trace developments in mostly English-language works on painting, sculpture, architecture, music, theater, and other disciplines. Instructional works on musical instruments, catalogs of art objects, comic operas, and more are also included.

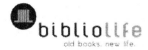

The BiblioLife Network

This project was made possible in part by the BiblioLife Network (BLN), a project aimed at addressing some of the huge challenges facing book preservationists around the world. The BLN includes libraries, library networks, archives, subject matter experts, online communities and library service providers. We believe every book ever published should be available as a high-quality print reproduction; printed on-demand anywhere in the world. This insures the ongoing accessibility of the content and helps generate sustainable revenue for the libraries and organizations that work to preserve these important materials.

The following book is in the "public domain" and represents an authentic reproduction of the text as printed by the original publisher. While we have attempted to accurately maintain the integrity of the original work, there are sometimes problems with the original work or the micro-film from which the books were digitized. This can result in minor errors in reproduction. Possible imperfections include missing and blurred pages, poor pictures, markings and other reproduction issues beyond our control. Because this work is culturally important, we have made it available as part of our commitment to protecting, preserving, and promoting the world's literature.

GUIDE TO FOLD-OUTS MAPS and OVERSIZED IMAGES

The book you are reading was digitized from microfilm captured over the past thirty to forty years. Years after the creation of the original microfilm, the book was converted to digital files and made available in an online database.

In an online database, page images do not need to conform to the size restrictions found in a printed book. When converting these images back into a printed bound book, the page sizes are standardized in ways that maintain the detail of the original. For large images, such as fold-out maps, the original page image is split into two or more pages

Guidelines used to determine how to split the page image follows:

• Some images are split vertically; large images require vertical and horizontal splits.
• For horizontal splits, the content is split left to right.
• For vertical splits, the content is split from top to bottom.
• For both vertical and horizontal splits, the image is processed from top left to bottom right.

THE
CHARTER

OF THE

ROYAL CANAL COMPANY,

K Dublin — Royal Canal Company

WITH THEIR

RULES,

AND

EXTRACTS FROM THE ACT OF THE 29th OF HIS
PRESENT MAJESTY GEORGE III.

WITH

AN INDEX.

TO WHICH IS PREFIXED,

A LIST OF THE SUBSCRIBERS.

DUBLIN:

PRINTED BY JOHN CHAMBERS, NO. 5, ABBEY-STREET.

M,DCC,LXXXIX.

SUBSCRIBERS NAMES.

HIS Grace the Duke of Leinster, £.1000
Right Hon. the Earl of Granard,   1000
Right Hon Lord Longford,   1000
Right Hon. Earl Carhampton,   600
Right Hon. Lord Sunderlin,   1000
Right Hon. Lord Viscount Ranelagh,   600
Right Hon. Lord Trimelston,   1000
Hon. Lord Delvin,   -   600
Rt. Hon. Sir John Blaquiere, K. B.   600
Right Hon. Thomas Conolly,   1000
Sir Will. Gleadowe Newcomen, Bart. 1800
Sir Thomas Fetherston, Bart.   1000
Sir Robert Hodson, Bart.   600
Hon. Robert Rochfort,   -   600
Hon Richard Annesley,   1200
Hon. Capt. Thomas Pakenham,   600
Robert Alexander, Esq.   -   600
Arthur Dawson, Esq.   -   600
John Hatch, Esq.   -   1000
Henry Cope, Esq.   -   1000
William Cope, Esq.   -   2000
John Binns, Esq.   -   2000
George Digby, Esq.   -   2000

a   Henry

SUBSCRIBERS NAMES.

Henry Stevens Riely, Efq.	£.2000
Randall M'Donnell, Efq.	2000
John Jones, Efq. - -	5000
John Giffard, Efq. -	2000
Mr. William Sinnett, -	2000
Mr. Michael Allen, - -	2000
James Napper Tandy, Efq.	2000
Mr. Charles Clark, -	2000
Mr. William Pike, -	2000
Thomas Tweedy, Efq. -	2000
Mr. William Crofby, -	2000
Pat. M'Loughlin, Efq. -	1000
Mr. John Copeland, -	1000
Arthur Riky, Efq, -	1000
Chriftopher Deey, Efq. -	1000
James Conolly, Efq. -	1000
Mrs. Ann Riely, - -	1000
Alexander Kirkpatrick, Efq.	1000
Mr. William Hauttenville,	1000
Thomas Andrews, Efq. -	1000
Mrs. Jane Hardin, - -	1000
Edward Bulkely, Efq. -	1000
Capt. John Pratt, -	1000
Mr. John Williams, -	1000
Mr. Peter Hoey, -	1000
Mr. Edward Clark, -	1000
Thomas Magan, Efq. -	1000
Mr. Nicholas Tallon, -	1000
Solomon Boileau, Efq. - -	1000
Richard Allen, Efq. -	1000
Robert Deey, Efq. - -	1000
William Shannon, Efq. -	1000
William Taylor, Efq, -	1000
James Fleming, Efq. -	1000

Charles

SUBSCRIBERS NAMES.

Charles Ward, Efq.	£ 1000
Charles Dillon Bellew, Efq.	1000
Mr. Thomas Dillon,	1000
Edward Whitten, Efq.	1000
Richard Cudmore, Efq.	1000
Mr. John Bufby,	1000
Mr. Henry Strong,	1000
Timothy Dyton, Efq.	1000
Thomas Walker, Efq.	1000
Mr. Daniel Finn,	1000
Mr. John Collins	1000
Major Jofeph Walker,	1000
Mr. George Binns,	900
Mrs. Elizabeth Archbold,	700
Sir James Nugent, Bart.	600
Sir Charles Levinge, Bart.	600
Thomas Tenifon, Efq.	600
Gafper Erck, Efq.	600
Capt. William Wright,	600
Mr. Andrew Gibbons,	600
Mr. John Crofthwaite,	600
Brent Nevill, Efq.	600
Mr. John Talbot,	600
John Allen, Efq.	600
Mr. William Twigg,	600
Sir Henry Jebb, Kt.	600
Rev. George Coates,	600
Charles Hamilton, Efq.	600
John Keogh, Efq.	600
Samuel Stock, Efq.	600
Rev. Meade Dennis,	600
Mr William Norris,	600
Mr. Charles Ryan,	600
Mr. Thomas Darcy,	600

Mr.

SUBSCRIBERS NAMES.

Mr. James Faucett,	£.600
Mr. Thomas Lynch,	600
Mr. Daniel Reily,	600
Henry Arabin, Efq.	600
Mrs. Mary Reily,	600
George Clibborn, Efq.	600
Mr. Clements Higginbotham,	600
Ben. Clarke, Efq.	600
William Fetherfton, Efq.	600
Mr. Ralph Mulhern,	600
Mark Anthony Blair, Efq.	600
Mr. Henry Hutton,	600
Mr. John Chambers,	600
Mr. Jofhua Dixon,	600
Mr. Robert Jofeph Shutter,	600
Rev. Henry Wynne,	600
John Riely, Efq	600
John Tyrrell, Efq.	600
Arthur Tyrrell, Efq.	600
Mr. James Henry,	600
Mr. Henry Jackfon,	600
Andrew Daly, Efq. M. D.	600
Francis Hopkins, Efq.	600
Charles Thorp, Efq.	600
Val. Dillon, Efq.	600
Mr. William Clarke,	600
Mr. James Dixon.	600
Robert Percival, Efq. M. D.	600
Mr. James Kelly,	600
Thomas Burrowes, Efq.	600
Mifs Mary Thewlefs	500
James Middleton Berry, Efq.	500
Mr. Samuel Downes,	500
Mrs. Mary Connor,	500

John

SUBSCRIBERS NAMES.

John Ladeveze, Esq.	£.500
John Verschoyle, Esq.	500
Mr. John Barber,	500
Joseph Donnelly, Esq.	500
Mr. Whitmore Davis,	400
Alderman Henry Gore Sankey,	300
Alderman William Alexander,	300
Alexander Lynar, Esq.	300
Mr. Nathaniel Caitland,	300
Mr. Charles Crosthwaite,	300
Captain Richard Chenevix	300
Riely Birmingham, Esq.	300
John Sankey, Esq.	300
Hartley Hodson, Esq.	300
Joseph Huband, Esq.	300
Mr. Ross Maguire,	300
John White, Esq.	300
Jasper Debrisay, Esq.	300
James Ormsby, Esq.	300
John Reynell, Esq.	300
Mr. Nicholas Le Favre,	300
Alexander Burrowes, Esq.	300
Mr. Thomas Hackett,	300
Mr. Philip Thomas Morpie,	300
Alexander Lindsay, Esq. M. D.	300
Captain John Daniel Arabin,	300
Ger. O'Ferral, Esq.	300
Mr. James Carey.	300
William Judge, Esq.	300
Robert Walsh, Esq	300
Mr. John Johnston,	300
Mr. John O'Brien,	300
Mr. Michael Doyle,	300
Mr. John Carey,	300

Mes-

SUBSCRIBERS NAMES.

Meſſdames C. and E. Fitzpatrick,	£.300
Mr. John Ward, - -	300
Mr. Samuel Ward, - -	300
Mr. Andrew Clark, - -	300
Mr. Walter Rooney, - -	300
Mr. Terence Duff, - -	300
Mr. Richard Fagan, - -	300
Mr. Mathias Flood, - -	300
Mr. James O'Brien, - -	300
Robert Ferrall, Eſq. - -	300
John Smith, Eſq. - -	300
Mr. Chriſtopher Carey, -	300
Charles O'Connor, Eſq. -	300
Myles Keon, Eſq. - -	300
Peter Delamare, Eſq. -	300
Mr. Thomas Hickey, - -	300
Mr. Bryan Kerin, - -	300
Mr. William Ruſſel, -	300
Mr. Henry Frazer, - -	300
Mr. John Ferral, - -	300
Mr. Patrick Byrne, - -	300
Mr. James Croſby, - -	300
Meſſrs James Farrel and William Davett, - - -	300
Arthur Brown, Eſq. Governor Kinſale, &c. - -	300
Mr. Patrick Corcoran, -	300
Miſs Letitia Veſey, - -	100
Mr. Nathaniel Low, - -	100
Mr. Thomas Shutter, - -	100
Mr. John Alder, - -	100
	£. 134,000

Subſcriptions,

SUBSCRIBERS NAMES.

Subfcriptions,   -   £. 134,000
Parliamentary Grant,   66,000

Fund of the Company £. 200,000

CHARTER

OF THE

ROYAL CANAL COMPANY.

GEORGE the Third, by the Grace of God, of Great Britain, France and Ireland King, Defender of the Faith and fo forth, To all unto whom thefe prefents fhall come, GREETING. WHEREAS Petition for the Charter. we are informed by the humble petition of our right trufty and right entirely beloved Coufin and Counfellor William Petioners Names. Robert Duke of Leinfter, our right trufty and right well beloved Coufin and Counfellor Henry Lawes Earl of Carhampton, our right trufty and well beloved Charles Lord Vifcount Ranelagh, our right trufty and well beloved Counfellor Edward Michael Lord Baron Longford, our right trufty and well beloved Richard Lord

B   Baron

Baron Sunderlin, our right trufty and well beloved Counfellor Sir John Blaquiere, Knight of the Bath, our trufty and well beloved Sir William Gleadowe Newcomen, Baronet, Sir Thomas Fetherfton, Baronet, John Hatch, Efq. Francis Fetherfton, Efq. William Alexander, Alderman, James Ormfby, Efq. Jafper Debrifay, Efq Captain William Wright, William Cope, Efq. John Binns, Efq. Thomas Andrews, Efq. and James Conolly, Efq. on behalf of themfelves and feveral other perfons, Undertakers for *To complete a Navigable Canal from Dublin to Tarmonbury on the Shannon* completing a Navigable Canal from Dublin to Tarmonbury, on the River Shannon, prefented to our Lord Lieutenant General and General Governor of our Kingdom of Ireland, That by an Act of Parliament, paffed in the laft Seffion of Parliament holden in our faid Kingdom of Ireland, entitled, " *An Act for the Promo-* *Act paffed to iffue 66,000l. in Debentures, at four per cent per ann.* " *tion and Encouragement of Inland Navi-* " *gation,*" it is amongft other things enacted, That debentures to the amount of 66,000l. bearing an intereft after the rate of 4l. per centum per annum, be iffued to fuch perfons as then were, or fhould be Undertakers for completing a Navigable Canal from Dublin to Tarmonbury, on the River Shannon, purfuant to their Petition prefented to the Houfe of Commons.

AND

AND the said Petitioners by their said petition set forth, that it is by the said Act enacted, That no debentures shall be issued, and that no grants shall be made to any such Undertakers as therein mentioned, unless such Undertakers shall actually have expended of their proper money on the Navigation under their management respectively, double the sum which they shall demand of the public money.

Provided double the sum of the public money be expended.

AND the said Petitioners by their said petition also set forth, That it is also thereby enacted, that so soon as any subscribers to any of the Undertakings therein mentioned, shall be constituted and created into a body corporate, they shall be and stand invested with, and shall hold and enjoy all and singular the like powers, privileges, advantages, and authorities in all things, for the purposes of carrying on the Navigation and Off-Branches therein mentioned, as were before the passing of the said Act vested in the Corporation for promoting and carrying on an Inland Navigation in Ireland, by virtue of the several Acts of Parliament heretofore passed in this kingdom, relative to and concerning Inland Navigation, and as were then vested by law in the Company of Undertakers of the Grand Canal, for the purpose of enabling them to carry on the said Canal.

And vesting like powers, &c with those of the Inland Navigation and Grand Canal Company

AND

Recital of the petition. AND the said Petitioners by their said petition also set forth, That the aforesaid petition mentioned in the said Act to have been presented to the House of Commons, was so presented by and on behalf of the said Petitioners, and several others who had then associated, and have since subscribed several sums of money for the purpose of carrying on and completing an Inland Navigation between the city of Dublin and the said town of Tarmonbury, on the River Shannon, in manner herein after mentioned.

AND the said Petitioners by their said petition also set forth, That until they and such other persons as have subscribed, and shall subscribe to the said Undertaking, shall be incorporated, the said Act will be to them inoperative, as they and the said Subscribers cannot, until they shall be so incorporated, be invested with any powers to proceed on the said Undertaking, or entitle themselves to the aid intended for them by the said Act.

Royal Grant. AND whereas our Lord Lieutenant General and General Governor of our said kingdom of Ireland, has laid before us, the said petitioners most humble request, that we would be graciously pleased by our Royal Charter, to constitute the said petitioners, and such other persons as have already subscribed, and may hereafter subscribe

subscribe to the said undertaking, a body corporate, for the purpose of carrying on the same, by the name of THE ROYAL CANAL COMPANY, with such powers, privileges, and authorities, as we in our royal wisdom shall think fit; and with which request of the said petitioners we are graciously pleased to comply.

KNOW YE THEREFORE, That we of our special grace certain knowledge and mere motion, by and with the advice and consent of our right trusty and right entirely beloved Counsellor Richard Baron Rokeby, Archbishop of Armagh, and Primate of all Ireland, our right trusty and well beloved Counsellor John Baron Fitzgibbon, our Chancellor of our said kingdom, and our right trusty and well beloved Counsellor John Foster, Speaker of the House of Commons of our said kingdom of Ireland, our Justices General and General Governors of our said kingdom of Ireland, and according to the tenor and effect of our Royal Letters, under our Privy Signet and Royal Sign Manual, bearing date at our Court at St. James's the 25th of August, 1789, *dated 25th Aug. 1789* and in the twenty-ninth year of our reign, and now enrolled in the Rolls of our High-Court of Chancery in our said kingdom of Ireland, HAVE made, ordained, authorized, constituted and appointed, and by these presents for us our heirs and successors,

succeffors, we do make, ordain, authorize, conftitute and appoint our right trufty and right entirely beloved Coufin and
Counfellor William Robert Duke of
Leinfter, our right trufty and right well beloved Coufin and Counfellor Henry Lawes
Earl of Carhampton, our right trufty and
well beloved Charles Lord Vifcount Ranelagh, our right trufty and well beloved
Counfellor, Edward Michael Lord Ba-
ron Longford our right trufty and well
beloved Richard Lord Baron Sunderlin,
our right trufty and well beloved Counfellor, Sir John Blaquiere, Knight of the
Bath, our trufty and well beloved Sir
William Gleadowe Newcomen, Baronet,
Sir Thomas Fetherfton, Bart. John Hatch,
Efq. Francis Fetherfton, Efq. William
Alexander, Alderman, James Ormfby,
Efq. Jafper Debrifay, Efq. Captain William Wright, William Cope, Efq. John
Binns, Efq. Thomas Andrews, Efq. and
James Conolly, Efq. and all fuch other
perfons as now have, or hereafter fhall
have any fhare or fhares in the joint ftock
herein after mentioned, to be one body
politic and corporate in deed and in name,
and to have continuance for ever, for the
purpofe of carrying on, and completing
the aforefaid Inland Navigation, between
the faid City of Dublin and the faid Town
of Tarmonbury, in manner herein after
mentioned, and for the making fuch Navigable Cuts and Off Branches, as herein
after

after mentioned, by the name of THE Stile and title
ROYAL CANAL COMPANY, and by
the fame name to have perpetual fuccef-
fion, and to fue and be fued, plead and By which to
be impleaded, anfwer and be anfwered fue and be
unto, defend and be defended, in all fued at law.
and whatfoever courts and places, and before any judges, juftices, or officers of
us, our heirs and fucceffors whatfoever,
in all and fingular actions, pleas, fuits,
plaints, matters and demands of what
kind or quality foever, they fhall be in
the fame manner and form, and as amply
as any of our fubjects, bodies politic or
corporate within our kingdom of Ireland;
and may have, purchafe, receive, take, To purchafe
poffefs, or enjoy all fuch lands, buildings or fell.
and appurtenances of what kind foever,
and alfo all fuch goods and chattels, as
fhall be neceffary, for making and pre-
ferving the faid Lines of Navigation, and
their Off-Branches; and may grant, alien,
demife, fell, or affign the fame, or any
part thereof, at their free will and pleafure; and to make and have a common One common
feal for them and their fucceffors, for the feal, change-
carrying on, and expediting the bufinefs able at plea-
and affairs of the faid Company, and for fure.
the enfealing, making and executing deeds,
grants, leafes and inftruments in writing
of what nature or kind foever, which they
fhall find neceffary to feal or make, relative to, or concerning any matter or thing
appertaining to the bufinefs of the faid
Company,

Company; and the same seal, at any time or times hereafter, to alter and change as they and their successors shall think fit.

Power to carry on and complete aforesaid Navigation, by two Canals

AND further, also we have given and granted, and by these presents for us, our heirs and successors, we do give and grant unto the said Company full power and authority by themselves, their agents, overseers, workmen, and servants, to carry on, and complete the aforesaid Navigation between the City of Dublin and the aforesaid Town of Tarmonbury, on the River Shannon, by means of two Canals, one of the said Canals to be cut and made from the River Liffey, near the

One Canal from New Custom-House The other Canal from Bolton-street.

New Custom-House, in Dublin, and the other of the said Canals to be cut and made from Bolton-Street, in the City of Dublin; each of the said Canals to be cut and made in such directions as that the

Both to unite near Prospect.

said two Canals shall unite near Prospect, on the road leading from Dublin to Glasnevin; which said Canal is from thence to be conducted to or near the said Town of

Great line of the Canal.

Tarmonbury, by a line to be carried on thro' or near Kilcock, Kinnegad, and Mullingar; and also to make a Navigable Cut from such part of the aforesaid line of Navigation, as may appear expedient, to,

Branch or branches from the main line

or towards the towns of Trim, Kells, Athboy, and Castletown-Delvin; and also to make and cut all such Navigable Off Branches from the said lines of Naviga-

tion

tion to fuch market-towns, or other places as may feem moft expedient.

AND our will and pleafure is, and we do hereby direct and appoint that the capital ftock of the faid Company fhall be the fum of 200,000l. that is to fay, the aforefaid fum of 66,000l. fo granted by the faid act, and the fum of 134,000l. to be fubfcribed as aforefaid. And that it fhall and may be lawful, to and for the faid Company, by any act or acts of the faid Company to be paff-ed at any general meeting, or meetings, to be held as herein after mentioned, to open any further fubfcription or fub-fcriptions, and thereby to raife any fur-ther fum or fums of money which they fhall find neceffary, not exceeding 300,000l. fterling, for the purpofe of car-rying on the faid work; which further fums when fubfcribed fhall be added to, and become a part of the joint ftock of the faid Company.

Capital Stock 200,000l.

66,000l. granted by Parliament. 134,000l. fubfcribed.

Which capi-tal may be enlarged by a fum not exceeding 300,000l.

AND our will and pleafure further is, and we do hereby alfo direct and appoint, that the feveral perfons who have fubfcribed and fhall fubfcribe to the faid Undertaking fhall, on or before the 10th day of November, 1789, pay into the hands of fuch perfon as fhall be appointed as Treafurer by the majority of the faid Company, to be affembled

Subfcribers to pay 5 per cent. of their refpective fubfcriptions by 10th No-vember, 1789, to the Treafurer.

for

for that purpofe, as herein after mentioned, 5l. per centum of the fums which ... ll be by them refpectively fubfcribed; ... default of fuch payment, the fub... ... of every perfon fo failing to pay ... ... folutely void to all intents and ... ... foever. And that the ... Company ... l receive other fubfcriptions for filling up fuch deficiency, until the fum of 134,000l. in the whole fhall be fubfcribed, and a depofit of 5l. per centum be made thereupon, as aforefaid.

Otherwife, their fubfcription to be void, the deficiency filled up

PROVIDED ALWAYS, that no perfon fhall be permitted to fubfcribe to the faid Undertaking lefs than the fum of 100l. And that no one perfon fhall be permitted to fubfcribe to the faid Undertaking either by himfelf or herfelf, or by any perfon or perfons in truft for him, or her, any greater fum, or to the amount of any greater fum, in the whole, than the fum of 5,000l. and that it fhall not at any time be lawful for any one perfon, either by himfelf or herfelf, or any perfon or perfons in truft for him or her, to purchafe, take, or acquire, or to have, or be in any manner poffeffed of, or entitled to, any greater fum, or to the amount of any greater fum, in the capital ftock of the faid Company, than the faid fum of 5,000l. in the whole: unlefs he or fhe fhall become entitled to

such

No original Subfcriber lefs than 100l.

Nor more than 5000l.

Unlefs poffeffed thereof by bequeft, or as executor or adminiftrator.

such overplus by bequest, or as executor or administrator of some person deceased. And that if any one person shall by any means whatsoever (save by bequest or as executor or administrator as aforesaid) either by himself or herself, or by any person or persons in trust for him or her, acquire or be in any manner possessed of any greater sum, or to the amount of any greater sum in the capital stock of the said Company, than the sum of 5,000l. in the whole; then, and in that case, such part of the said stock as such persons shall so acquire, or be possessed of, over and above the said sum of 5,000l. shall be forfeited for the benefit of the said Company. And that it shall and may be lawful, to and for the said Company, to sell and dispose of the same by public cant, and to apply the money arising by such sale to the purposes of the said Undertaking.

Any person becoming possessed of more than 5000l. except by bequest or as executor or administrator, shall forfeit the same to the Company, and be disposed of by public cant.

AND our will and pleasure further is, and we do hereby order, direct, and appoint, that the joint stock of the said Company shall be divided into shares of 100l. each.

Joint stock divided into shares of 100l. each.

AND our will and pleasure further is, and we do hereby ordain and appoint, that the said Company, and their successors shall, in every year, hold four certain General Assemblies, or meetings, of

Four annual stated general meetings, 1st Feb. 11th May, 15th July, 15th Nov.

of the said Company, that is to say, on every 1st day of February, 1st day of May, 15th day of July, and 15th day of November, unless any of the said days should happen on a Sunday, and in such case, that the meeting shall be held on the following day. And shall also have full power and authority at all other times as occasion shall require, to assemble in the city of Dublin, and from time to time to adjourn such assemblies, and at such assemblies, or any adjournment thereof, under the directions and regulations hereafter mentioned, to make such by-laws for the better government of the said Corporation; and for making such contracts or agreements, and such rules and orders, as may be necessary for carrying on the said Navigation; and appointing such engineers, overseers, and other persons for carrying on and conducting the business of the said Navigation, as they shall think fit. Which by-laws, rules, or orders, being passed and agreed to at any assembly of the said Company, or at any adjournment thereof, by a majority of the members of the said Company present at such assembly, or adjournment, and qualified to vote thereat as herein after is mentioned, shall be valid and binding upon the said Company and the members thereof, and upon all persons employed by them. And that the said Company shall at such
assemblies,

Any of said days falling on a Sunday, to be held on the following day.

At all other times may meet in Dublin, to make by-laws or other regulations.

By-laws or other regulations made by the majority of a legal assembly, binding on said Company and dependents.

By-laws &c. may also be amended or

affemblies, or adjournments thereof, and by a majority of the perfons then prefent, qualified as aforefaid, have full power and authority to alter, vary, and amend fuch by-laws, rules, and orders, or any of them, as they fhall think fit: provided always, that fuch by-laws, rules, and orders, fhall not be contrary to the laws or ftatutes of our faid kingdom of Ireland. *annulled at any of faid meetings.*

But no by-law, rule, or order, to be made contrary to the laws of the realm.

AND our will and pleafure further is, and we do hereby order, direct, and appoint, that feven days notice at the leaft, including the day of fuch notice, and the day of holding any affembly of the faid Company, (fave the aforefaid four ftated affemblies, and fuch affemblies as fhall be held by adjournment) fhall be given of the time and place of holding fuch affembly, in fuch public News-paper of the city of Dublin, as fhall be agreed on by the faid Company. Save only, that when any fuch affembly fhall be intended to be held for the purpofe of choofing and electing directors of the faid Company, or of appointing any officer to the faid Company; or for taking into confideration the difmiffal of any officer of the faid Company; or any complaint againft any fuch officer; or for the purpofe of taking into confideration any contract to be made relative to the faid Navigation, or the works there-of; *Seven days notice of holding any fuch meetings (except the four general ftated meetings, or adjourned meetings) to be given in a Dublin public News-paper.*

But if a meeting is to be held for electing directors, or other officers, or for difmiffal of, or complaint againft any officer, or relative to any contract or work to be carried on, for borrowing money or disposing of any property, or for reward of any person, then fourteen days notice in two public Dublin Newspapers, to be given.

of; or the borrowing of money, or letting or disposing of any of the estates or property of the said Company; or for the taking into consideration the carrying on any work or works appertaining to the aforesaid undertaking; or the rewarding any person or persons for any particular service or services; then, and upon any of the said last mentioned occasions, fourteen days notice at the least

No new business to be entered on at any adjourned meeting.

shall be given in two of the public Newspapers which shall be then published in the said city of Dublin; and that at any adjourned meeting, no new business shall be proposed or entered upon.

No person qualified to vote unless he have three shares of capital stock of 100l. each.

PROVIDED ALWAYS, and we do hereby direct and declare our will and pleasure to be, that no person shall be permitted or qualified to vote at any assembly of the said Company, or any adjournment thereof, or have any right to intermeddle in any sort in the affairs of the said Company, unless he or she shall have, in his or her own name and right, or in right of his or her testator, or intestate, at least

Nor then to have more than one vote, which vote may be given personally, or by proxy.

three shares of the stock of the said Company of 100l. each; and that no Member of the said Company shall have more than one vote at each of the assemblies of the said Company; and that every Member who shall have a right to vote at such assemblies, may appear either in person

A vote by proxy to be

or by proxy; such proxy being also a
Member

Member of the faid Company having a under the right to vote, and to be appointed by an hand and inftrument in writing, under the hand feal of the and feal of the perfon appointing fuch perfon deputing. proxy.

AND our will and pleafure further is, Any body politic or corpoand we do hereby ordain and direct, that litic or corporate, poffeffin cafe any body-politic or corporate, ing three fhall at any time become poffeffed of, or fhares of entitled to three or more fhares of the 100l. each, ftock of the faid Company of 100l. each, may appoint, it fhall be lawful for fuch body politic or under feal, corporate, by inftrument in writing under a proxy, who may act as their corporate feal, to appoint any per- one of the fon to vote on the part of fuch body po- Members litic or coporate at fuch affemblies as aforefaid; and that it fhall be lawful for the perfon who fhall be fo appointed, to give one vote on the part of fuch body politic or corporate at every fuch affembly, and in all refpects to act as the other Members of the faid Company.

PROVIDED ALSO, and we do hereby No perfon direct and appoint, that after the expira- poffeffed of tion of twelve months, to be computed fhares by affignment from the time when the aforefaid fubfcrip- or transfer, tion fhall be filled and completed, no before 12 perfon whatever fhall be qualified or per- months be mitted to vote at any affembly or meeting completing of the faid Company, upon or by virtue the original of any affignment or transfer from any fubfcription, other perfon or perfons of any fhare or and that the fame be enfhares tered in the

transfer book shares of the stock of the said Company,
6 months, is unless such assignment or transfer shall
qualified to have been really and actually made and
vote. entered in the transfer-book of the said
Company, for the full space of six calendar months, previous to the time of his
or her tendering such vote or votes.

But not to   PROVIDED ALWAYS, that such regula-
affect persons tion shall not extend to, or affect any
who become person or persons who shall become pof-
poffeffed by feffed of, or entitled to any share or shares
bequeft, or as
executors or of the said stock by bequeft, or as execu-
adminiftra- tor or adminiftrator.
tors.

No perfon to   AND PROVIDED ALSO, and we do here-
give more by direct, ordain and declare, that no
than two Member of the said Company shall at any
votes as the
proxy of any affembly of the said Company, give more
Member or than two votes as the proxy of any other
Members. Member or Members of the said Company.

No perfon to   AND our will and pleasure further is,
vote as proxy and we do hereby direct, ordain and ap-
unless an en-
try of fuch point, that before any perfon shall be per-
proxy be mitted to vote in any affembly of the said
previoufly Company, under any proxy which shall
made in the
Secretary's be granted by any Member of the said
book, con- Company, an entry of such proxy shall
taining the be made in a book to be kept by the Se-
names of the
perfon grant- cretary of the said Company for that pur-
ing and to pofe; which entry shall contain the date
whom grant- of such proxy, and the name of the per-
ed, with the
date thereof. fon

son granting the same; and also the name
of the person to whom the same shall be
granted.   And that no person whatever,
save the person named as proxy in such
entry, shall be permitted to vote as proxy
for the person granting the proxy which
shall be so entered.   And that no more
than one proxy shall be entered at the
same time in the said book.   And that in
case the person granting such proxy shall
afterwards grant a second proxy to any
other person, such second proxy shall not
be voted under, or be of any force or
effect, until the same shall be entered in
the said book.   And that from the time
of the entry of such second proxy in the
said book, the proxy which shall have
been so first entered, shall become ab-
solutely null and void to all intents and
purposes, and so from time to time as to
all subsequent proxies, which shall be
granted by any Member of the said
Company, the last of which proxies,
which shall be so entered in the said book,
shall supersede and render null and void
all former proxies granted by the person
granting such last proxy; so as that no
more than one person, shall at any one
time be impowered to vote as proxy, for
any Member of the said Company, any
reservation, proviso, or contingency,
contained or expressed, or to be contained or expressed in any such proxy, in any
wise notwithstanding.

But if the person granting such proxy afterward issue another to a different person, this last, before of any effect, to be also entered as the foregoing, when the former becomes null; and so of every subsequent change.

C   AND

AND our will and pleasure is, and we do hereby direct, ordain and declare, that no person shall be qualified or permitted to vote in his own right, in any assembly or meeting of the said Company, who shall not, at such assembly or meeting, if thereto required by any Member of the said Company then present, (having a right to vote) take the following oath, (or, if of the people called Quakers, affirmation) before the Chairman, who shall preside at such assembly or meeting; and which oath or affirmation the said Chairman is hereby empowered to administer: that is to say,

No person qualified to vote unless, if required at the time, he take the prescribed oath before the Chairman.

The Oath of a Member

" *I* (*A. B.*) *do swear* (or *being of*
" *the people called Quakers, do affirm*),
" *that I am now possessed of*
"
" *capital stock, in the*
" *Royal Canal Company, in my own right,*
" *or as executor or administrator of* (*C. D.*)
" *deceased; and that I do not hold the same,*
" *or any part thereof, directly or indirectly*
" *in trust for any other person or persons;*
" *and that I have not any confidence or ex-*
" *pectation, nor have I entered into any agree-*
" *ment, expressed or implied, that the person*
" *or persons from whom I purchased or ac-*
" *quired the same, will return to me, direct-*
" *ly or indirectly, the consideration or security*
" *which I gave for the said stock, upon my*
" *assigning the same to him, her, or them, or*
" *for his, her or their use. And that I did*
' *not purchase or acquire the said stock, or*
" *any part thereof, with any intention of*
" *re-assigning*

" re affigning the fame, or any part thereof,
" directly or indirectly, to any perfon or
" perfons, from whom I purchafed or acquir-
" ed the fame, or to any other perfon or per-
" fons for his, her, or their ufe "

AND our will and pleafure is, and we No perfon to vote by proxy unlefs, if re-quired at the time, to take the prefcrib-ed oath. do hereby direct, ordain, and declare, that no perfon fhall be qualified or per-mitted, at any meeting of the faid Com-pany, to vote by virtue of any proxy or proxies granted to him, or her, by any perfon or perfons, unlefs the perfon or perfons tendering fuch vote or votes, un-der fuch proxy or proxies, fhall (if there-to required by any Member of the faid Company then prefent having a right to vote) take the following oath, or if of the people called Quakers, affirmation, before the Chairman, who fhall prefide at fuch affembly or meeting; and which oath or affirmation the faid Chairman is hereby empowered to adminifter: that is to fay,

" I (A. B.) do fwear, or affirm, that The oath of a proxy " I verily believe that (C D.) the per- " fon for whom I now vote as proxy, is pof- " feffed in his, or her own right, or as execu- " tor or adminiftrator of (C. D.) (as the " cafe may be) of the ftock mentioned in the " proxy by virtue of which I vote."

AND our will and pleafure further is, Every perfon granting a proxy at figning the inftrument to and we do hereby direct, ordain and de-clare, that every perfon who fhall fign

C 2

make oath before a Justice of Peace.

an inftrument of proxy, to enable another to vote for him or her, fhall, at the
time of figning fuch inftrument, make,
before any of our Juftices of Peace, an
affidavit, or, if of the people called Quakers, affirmation, to be annexed to fuch
inftrument in the words following.

The oath of a granter of a proxy.

" I (A. B.) do fwear, or affirm, that I
" was, at the time of figning the annexed
" inftrument of proxy, and that I now am
" poffeffed of the capital ftock in the faid in-
" ftrument of proxy mentioned, in my own
" right, as executor or adminiftrator of (A.
" B.) or (C. D.) deceafed, (as the cafe may
" be) and that I do not hold the fame, or any
" part thereof, directly or indirectly, in truft
" for any other perfon or perfons, and that
" I have not entered into any agreement, ex-
" preffed or implied, nor have I any confi-
" dence or expectation, that the perfon or per-
" fons from whom I purchafed or acquired
" the fame will return to me, directly or in-
" directly, the confideration or fecurity which
" I gave for the faid ftock, upon my affigning
" the fame to him, her, or them, for his,
" her, or their ufe; and that I did not pur-
" chafe or acquire the faid ftock, or any part
" thereof, with any intention of re-affigning
" the fame, or any part thereof, directly or
" indirectly, to any perfon or perfons from
" whom I purchafed or acquired the fame, or
" any other perfon or perfons, for his, her,
" or their ufe; and that I will, upon my
" ceafing

" *ceafing to poffefs the faid flock, inform the*
" *Secretary of the faid Company thereof, if*
" *required by him fo to do.*" And which
oath fuch Juftice or Juftices of the Peace is
and are hereby empowered to adminifter.

AND our will and pleafure is, and we
do hereby direct and ordain, that no
perfon voting by proxy from any perfon
reprefenting any body politic or corporate, fhall be required to take the aforefaid oaths, or any of them, fo far as fuch
perfon fhall vote in right of fuch repre-
fentation.

No proxy of a body politic or corporate obliged to take any of aforefaid oaths.

AND we do hereby further direct, ordain and appoint, that a majority of votes
at fuch affemblies, and all adjournments
thereof, fhall determine all matters in
queftion before the faid Company; and
if there fhall be an equality of votes, that
the Chairman of fuch affemblies refpectively fhall have a cafting vote, befides
his vote as a Member of the faid Company.

A majority of votes to determine; but on equality the Chairman a cafting vote.

AND our will and pleafure further is,
and we do hereby ordain, direct and
appoint, that to conftitute a meeting of
the faid Company, of which feven days
notice only fhall be neceffary to be given
as aforefaid, there fhall be prefent in perfon nine Members at the leaft, who fhall
have a right to vote under the regulations
herein

Nine Members a legal meeting, with 7 days notice.

Thirteen Members a legal meeting with 14 days notice.

herein contained. And that to constitute a meeting of the said Company, of which fourteen days notice shall be necessary to be given as aforesaid, there shall be present in person thirteen persons at the least, who shall have a right to vote as aforesaid, or otherwise that such meetings respectively shall not have any power to act.

The accounts to be regularly kept in books to which every possessor of three shares may have access

AND we do hereby further direct, ordain and appoint, that the accounts, transactions, and proceedings of the said Company shall be fairly and regularly entered in books to be kept for that purpose, to which every person, having in his own name and right, or as executor or administrator to any person, three shares of one hundred pounds each, in such joint stock; and any person representing any body-politic or corporate as aforesaid, may have access at all reasonable times to inspect the same.

The company to receive from every vessel a rate not exceeding 3d a mile for every ton weight of cargo.

AND we do hereby for us, our heirs and successors, direct, declare, ordain and appoint, that in consideration of the expence and trouble which the said Company shall be put to in making and maintaining the said Navigation, together with the Off-Branches thereof, it shall and may be lawful, to and for the said Company, and their successors, from time to time, and at all times hereafter, to ask, demand, receive and sue, for the use of the

said

said Company, the several rates and duties herein after mentioned: that is to say, For every boat, barge, or other vessel navigating the said Canal, or any part thereof, either upwards or downwards, in which any goods, merchandizes, or commodities, or other matter whatsoever shall be carried, such rates and duties as the said Company shall ordain and appoint, not exceeding the sum of three-pence for every mile, for every ton of the burthen or tonage of such barge or other vessel, or for every ton weight of such goods, merchandizes, commodities, or other matter whatsoever, which shall be carried upwards or downwards, at the discretion of the said Company. And for each passenger in any such vessel, any sum not exceeding the sum of two-pence for every mile such passenger shall be carried. And an additional rate, not exceeding two-pence per ton, for every lock any such vessel shall pass through the communication of the said Navigation, between the junctions of the aforesaid Canals at Glassnevin road aforesaid and the River Liffey. Save and except, and provided always, that no higher toll than three-half-pence per mile be charged on each ton weight of corn, meal, malt, or flour brought to Dublin by the said Navigations.

And for every Passenger in such vessel at a Rate not exceeding 2d a mile.

And an additional rate not exceeding 2d. a ton for every lock such vessel shall pass, between the junction of the Canals at Glassnevin Road and the Liffey.

But corn, meal, &c. brought to Dublin, no higher toll than 1½d. a mile.

AND

No duty or cuſtom but thoſe taken as aforeſaid by the Company ſhall be taken for or upon any goods carried by ſaid Canal.

AND further alſo, we do hereby order, ordain and appoint, that no duty, rate, toll or cuſtom whatſoever, ſave the rates herein mentioned to be taken by the ſaid Company, ſhall be taken by the ſaid Company for, upon, or out of any goods, merchandizes, commodities, or other matter whatſoever, which ſhall or may be carried by the ſaid Canal to or for any place whatſoever.

Proprietors of ſaid joint ſtock entitled to profits in proportion to their reſpective intereſts in ſaid ſtock.

AND further alſo, we do hereby direct, ordain and appoint, that the proprietors of the ſaid joint ſtock, their executors, adminiſtrators and aſſigns, ſhall be entitled to the tolls, duties, advantages and profits hereby veſted in the ſaid Company, in proportion to their reſpective intereſts in the ſaid joint ſtock of the ſaid Company, ſubject to ſuch charges as the ſaid Company ſhall think fit to make for the completing and preſerving the ſaid works, and to the ſoil and water of the Canals, together with the banks thereof, and ſuch other portions of ground as the ſaid Company are impowered to acquire by virtue hereof.

Every proprietor of joint ſtock may bequeath or aſſign the ſame, but

AND we do hereby alſo direct, ordain and appoint, that it ſhall and may be lawful for every proprietor of ſuch joint ſtock to bequeath the ſame, or to aſſign the ſame in his life-time, and that every aſſignment which ſhall be made of any

part

part of the joint stock, shall be entered and made in a book for that purpose to be kept, at such place as shall be appointed by the said Company, and to be called the Transfer Book; and that no assignment shall be deemed good until entry be made in such book as aforesaid.

shall not be deemed valid until entry thereof be made in the Company's transfer book.

AND we do hereby also further direct, ordain and declare, that it shall and may be lawful to and for the said meetings, convened as herein before directed, from time to time, and at such times as may be necessary, to require the several proprietors of the said joint stock, to pay in such parts of their respective subscriptions as the said meetings shall think necessary for carrying on the said works; provided always, that no greater sum than twenty pounds per cent. on the several original subscriptions shall be required to be paid in any one year. And that in case any of the proprietors of the said joint stock, their representatives or assigns, shall refuse or neglect to pay the sum so called for, within thirty days after the time appointed by such meetings for the payment thereof, notice shall be given in two public newspapers in the city of Dublin, that the said Company will proceed to sell by public cant, on such days as shall be specified in such notice, the share or shares of the person or persons so refusing or neglecting to pay the sum or sums which

The proprietors of said joint stock may be required, by a meeting, to pay in such proportions of their original Subscriptions, not exceeding 20 per cent in one year, as shall be judged necessary.

But if such Proprietors shall not pay in the sums required within the limitations specified, then their shares to be sold by public cant, and the profits accruing to vest in the purchasers.

they

they fhall have been required to pay, and unlefs fuch perfon or perfons fhall before the day fpecified in fuch notice pay the refpective fums fo required to the faid Company, or fuch perfons as they fhall appoint for the purpofe, the faid Company fhall fell by public cant at the ufual place of the faid Company's meeting, the fhare or fhares of the perfon or perfons fo refufing to pay, and the money for which the fame fhall be fold fhall be paid to the faid Company, for the ufe of fuch proprietor or proprietors. And fuch proprietor or proprietors from thenceforth fhall be for ever barred from fuch fhare or fhares, and all profits arifing therefrom, and of all intereft in the fame, both in law or equity; and fuch fhare or fhares, and all profits and advantages arifing therefrom, fhall from thenceforth be vefted in fuch purchafer or purchafers.

And our will and pleafure further is, and we do hereby direct and appoint, that fuch notice fhall be given at leaft thirty days previous to the fale, including the day of fuch notice and the day of fale.

The clear profits to be divided among the Proprietors

And we do hereby alfo further direct and appoint, that the clear profits which fhall arife to the faid Company from the feveral duties hereby vefted in them, or otherwife,

otherwife, or fo much thereof as fhall be thought proper, fhall, from time to time, at Lady Day and at Michaelmas, or within fifteen days after the faid feafts refpectively, be divided and paid to and amongft the refpective proprietors of the faid joint ftock, in proportion to their feveral and refpective fhares and interefts therein.

in proportion to their refpective fhares and interefts, half yearly

And that if the faid Company fhall have occafion at any time to borrow money for carrying on the faid works, it fhall be lawful for the faid Company to take up and borrow upon the credit of the faid works and their eftate therein, or upon any annuity or annuities, for one or more life or lives to be charged upon the fame, or the aforefaid tolls, rates, and duties, any fum not exceeding the amount of the fubfcriptions actually expended on faid works, at any rate of intereft not exceeding legal intereft, and to ftrike debentures for fuch fum fo borrowed, in fuch manner as faid Company fhall appoint; which debentures, or life annuities, fhall be an actual charge and lien upon fuch parts of the faid Company's eftate as fhall be therein fpecified.

The Company may, borrow any fum not exceeding the amount of the fubfcriptions expended on faid works, at an intereft not exceeding the legal, and ftrike Debentures for the fame

And, laftly, we do declare and ordain, that thefe our letters patent, and every claufe, fentence and article therein contained, or the enrollment thereof, fhall be in all things firm, valid, fufficient and effectual

Charter to be enrolled in the court of Chancery within fix months from 1ft October, 1789

fectual in the law unto the said Company, according to the purport and tenor thereof, without any further grant, licence, or toleration from us, our heirs or successors, to be procured or obtained.

PROVIDED ALWAYS, that these our Letters Patent be enrolled in the Rolls of our High Court of Chancery, in our said kingdom of Ireland, within the space of six months from the date hereof, otherwise these our Letters Patent to be null, void, and of no effect, any thing herein contained to the contrary in anywise notwithstanding.

IN witness whereof we have caused these our Letters to be made Patent. WITNESS our aforesaid Justices General and General Governors of our said kingdom of Ireland, at Dublin the first day of October, in the twenty-ninth year of our Reign.

O'BRIEN.

(SEAL.)

(*Enrolled the 24th October,* 1789)

RULES

OF THE

ROYAL CANAL COMPANY.

THAT for the better managing the affairs of the Company, and establishing a continual succession of persons to be Directors thereof, a general assembly of the Company shall meet within one calendar month from the day of the date of their incorporation, fourteen days notice being first given of the said meeting. And that the Company shall, at such assembly, proceed to elect and choose from among the Members thereof, and by a majority of votes of the Members of the Company then present in person, or by proxy, forty-one persons to be directors; each of which persons shall be possessed of and intitled unto six hundred pounds at

the

A general meeting within one month after incorporation, giving 14 days notice thereof.

To chuse 41 persons as Directors, possessed of at least 600l. stock, each

the leaſt of the capital ſtock of the Company; which ſaid forty-one Directors ſo

elected and choſen, ſhall continue in office as Directors, from the time of ſuch
election until others ſhall be duly choſen
in their reſpective places; unleſs they, or
any of them, ſhall ſooner die, reſign, or
become diſqualified.

And that in each and every year for
ever thereafter, a general aſſembly of the
Company ſhall meet on ſome day in the
month of January in every year, fourteen
days previous notice of ſuch meeting
being given; and ſhall in like manner
elect and chooſe from among the Members of the Company, and by the majority
of votes of the Members of the Company
then preſent, either in perſon or by
proxy, forty-one perſons, to be Directors
of the Company for the year then next
enſuing; each of which perſons ſhall be
poſſeſſed of ſix hundred pounds at the leaſt
of the ſaid capital ſtock, and which ſaid

forty-one perſons ſo to be annually choſ-
en, ſhall ſeverally continue in office for
one year, from the time of ſuch their
election, and until others ſhall be duly
choſen into their places reſpectively; unleſs in caſe of death, reſignation, or diſ-
qualification.

That the ſaid forty-one perſons ſo to
be choſen and elected, or any five or

more

more of them, fhall be called A COURT OF DIRECTORS, for the ordering, managing and directing the affairs of the Company; and fhall, under the rules, orders and regulations of the Company, carry on, conduct and tranfact the general bufinefs of the Company : fubject neverthelefs to the control of the Company.

THAT no perfon fhall continue in office as a director longer than he fhall be poffeffed, in his own name and right, of fix hundred pounds at the leaft in the capital ftock of the faid Company; but that upon parting with fo much of his fhare in the faid ftock as may reduce the fame to any leffer fum than fix hundred pounds, the office of fuch Director fhall ceafe and become vacant, and another Director fhall be chofen in his room by the Company, in manner aforefaid.

THAT in cafe of the death, refignation, or difqualification of any of the faid Directors for the time being, the furvivors of them, or the majority of thofe remaining in office, fhall, within one month of fuch death, refignation, or difqualification of any of the faid Directors, call an affembly of the Company, in order to elect, and the Company fhall at fuch affembly elect another perfon, or other perfons qualified as aforefaid, in the room of the perfon or

perfons

perfons who fhall die, refign, or become difqualified.

That until a dividend fhall be made of the profits which fhall arife to the Company from the faid Undertaking, the feveral fubfcribers fhall, out of the property of the Company, be paid legal intereft for the fums which fhall be by them refpectively advanced, from the time of their advancing the fame refpectively, fuch intereft to be paid half yearly, at Lady-day and Michaelmas in every year, until fuch dividend of the faid profits fhall be made among the faid fubfcribers. And that from and after the making of fuch dividend, the faid intereft fhall ceafe and be no longer payable.

PROVIDED that the funds of the Company fhall not, by payment of fuch intereft, be at any time reduced to a leffer fum than that directed by Act of Parliament to be fubfcribed and raifed for faid Undertaking to intitle the Company to the aid of 66,000l. provided for them by the faid Act. And that no payment, on account of fuch intereft, fhall be brought into any account of expenditure which may be laid before the Commiffioners of Impreft Accounts, for the purpofe of claiming any part of faid aid.

THAT no perſon ſhall be elected into any office or employment under the Company, until the ſaid Court of Directors ſhall have firſt reported to the Company their opinion, after due examination, that ſuch perſon appears to them to be eligible for the office for which he ſhall propoſe himſelf as a candidate.

No perſon to be elected into office, until Court of Directors report to Company their eligibility.

THAT no Member of the Company, who ſhall qualify himſelf to vote in the meetings or aſſemblies of the ſaid Company, or grant a proxy to any perſon to vote for him, ſhall enter into or be in any manner, directly or indirectly, concerned in any contract with the Company, or hold any lucrative office or employment whatever under the Company, or enter into ſecurity to the Company for any officer or contractor.

No Member to enter into any contract with the Company, or hold any lucrative office, or be ſecurity for ſuch.

AND that no officer of the Company ſhall enter into, or be in any manner, directly or indirectly, concerned in any contract, or enter into any ſuch ſecurity as aforeſaid, ſave ſuch ſecurity as ſuch officer may enter into for the faithful performance of the office or employment which he ſhall hold under the Company.

No officer of the Company to enter into, or be concerned in any ſuch contract or ſecurity.

THAT the Company, at their firſt general meeting, ſhall determine on the two newſpapers they will advertize in.

Firſt general meeting to appoint the two Newspapers for advertiſing

D THE

Proceedings of former meeting first read and and signed at subsequent one.

THAT at all meetings of the Company, or Court of Directors, the proceedings of the last meeting shall be first read, and signed by the Chairman.

No Member to be present when business anywise concerning him, is immediately before the assembly.

THAT when any Member of the Company, or Court of Directors, is personally interested in any matter depending before the Company or Court of Directors, he shall withdraw whilst that subject is under consideration.

The books to be properly Index'd.

THAT the books of the Company, and Court of Directors, shall have an index, by which reference may be easily had to every transaction.

Work to be executed every year, to be estimated at commencement, that expences may equalize income.

THAT prior to the commencement of the works in every year, the Company shall determine what length of navigation shall be executed in the ensuing year: so soon as they shall ascertain the amount of the expence thereof, by the contracts necessary to be entered into for its completion. And that the sums expended in each year shall, as nearly as possible, equalize the income of the Company.

Depository for seal, &c. keys of which left by three Members.

THAT a proper Repository shall be provided for the Seal of the Company; and for deeds, maps, sections, and all papers of consequence, with three locks, the keys of which shall be deposited with three Members, to be chosen annually by the

the Company, when the Directors are elected.

THAT no deed, map, section, or other paper of consequence, shall be permitted to be taken out of the Company's house, without a receipt be given for the same, in a book kept for that purpose.

No deed, map, &c. taken, without receipt entered in the book

THAT the Charter and Rules of the Company be printed for the information of the Members.

Charter and Rules to be printed.

EXTRACTS

FROM

An Act of Parliament for the Promotion and Encouragement of Inland Navigation paſſed in Ireland, *Anno Regni Viceſimo Nono Georgii* III. *Regis.*

Printed by Permiſſion of His Majeſty's Printer.

" AND be it further enacted, that Debentures to the amount of ſixty-ſix thouſand pounds, bearing an intereſt after the rate of four pounds per centum per annum, be iſſued to ſuch perſons as are, or ſhall be Undertakers for completing a Navigable Canal from Dublin to Tarmonbury on the River Shannon, purſuant to their petition preſented to the Houſe of Commons this Seſſion of Parliament,

66,000l. to iſſue in Debentures at 4 per cent. per ann. as herein.

ment, subject to the several conditions, limitations, and restrictions herein after mentioned."

Said debentures not to be issued before 25 Mar. 1790, for greater sum in the whole than 25,000l.

" AND be it further enacted, That such debentures shall not be issued before the twenty-fifth day of March, one thousand seven hundred and ninety, for any greater sum in the whole than twenty-five thousand pounds; and after the twenty-fifth day of March, one thousand seven hundred and

nor for more than 25,000l in any year after;

ninety, that such debentures shall not be issued in any one year for the purposes herein mentioned, for any greater sum than the sum of twenty-five thousand

in case of application for more than 25,000l. in one year, those first applying to have priority in the year succeeding.

pounds in the whole, but in case application shall be made within any one year for debentures, exceeding in the whole such sum of twenty-five thousand pounds by persons entitled under this act to receive the same, such persons so applying, shall be entitled to receive such debentures in the subsequent year, according to the priority of time in which such applications for debentures were made by them respectively."

Lord Lieutenant may authorize the Vice Treasurers to issue debentures for a further sum

" PROVIDED always, That it shall and may be lawful for the Lord Lieutenant General, or other Chief Governor of this kingdom for the time being, to authorize the Vice-Treasurer or Vice-Treasurers, Paymaster or Paymasters-General, his or their Deputy or Deputies, to issue deben-

tures

tures for a further sum in any one year, not exceeding ten thousand pounds."

not exceed-
ing 10,000l.
in any year.

" PROVIDED always, and be it enacted, That no debentures shall be issued, and that no such grants shall be made to any such Subscribers, Undertakers, or Bodies Corporate, unless such Subscribers, Undertakers, or Bodies Corporate, shall actually have expended of their proper money on the navigation under their management respectively double the sum which they shall demand of the public money, and such Subscribers, Undertakers, or Bodies Corporate respectively, shall not be entitled to receive a debenture or debentures for any sum of the public money, until proof shall be made by or on behalf of such Subscribers, Undertakers, or Bodies Corporate respectively, before the Commissioners of Imprest Accounts of the expenditure of a sum amounting to double the sum for which such Subscribers, Undertakers, or Bodies Corporate respectively, shall demand one or more debentures pursuant to this act, it being the true intent and meaning of this act, that such Subscribers, Undertakers, or Bodies Corporate respectively, shall actually have expended of their proper money, a sum in the proportion of two-thirds for one-third which they shall receive of the public money, and such Subscribers, Undertakers, or Bodies Corporate

Provided
that subscri-
bers have ex-
pended of
their own
money dou-
ble what
they apply
for;

proof to be
made before
Commission-
ers of Im-
prest Ac-
counts of
such expen-
diture,

the intention
being, that
such compa-
nies shall ex-
pend 2 3ds
of their pro-
per money
for 1-3d of
the public
money,

and shall also prove before said Commissioners the expenditure of the 1-3d. before receiving any debenture for the same.

porate respectively, shall prove before the said Commissioners of Imprest Accounts, the expenditure of said one-third part for which one or more debentures shall have issued as aforesaid, before they shall be entitled to receive any debenture pursuant to this act, upon any further application for carrying on, or completing such works.

Bodies corporate entitled to any benefit under this Act, to deposite in National Bank 1-10th part of their subscriptions, or Government Securities for the same, and be entitled to the interest on securities so deposited, such deposite to be made in 18 months after 24 June 1789

"AND be it enacted, that all bodies corporate, who are entitled to any benefit under this Act, shall deposite with the Governor and Company of the Bank of Ireland, who are hereby required to receive the same, one-tenth part of their respective subscriptions or government securities for such tenth part, such subscriptions respectively being double the sum for which such bodies corporate respectively are by this Act entitled to receive debentures, and such bodies corporate, depositing such government securities, shall be entitled to receive the interest payable on the same, so long as they shall remain deposited in the said Bank, which deposite shall be made by such bodies corporate respectively, within eighteen calendar months after the twenty-fourth day of June next."

Bodies corporate expending any sum in carrying on

"PROVIDED ALWAYS, and be it enacted, that if such bodies corporate respectively, shall within the said eighteen months, actually expend any sum in the

carryin

carrying on such works, and prove such expenditure before the said Commissioners of Impress Accounts, such bodies corporate shall have credit for, and be entitled to so much in their respective deposites, and such bodies corporate shall after the expiration of six calendar months from the twenty-fourth day of June next, be entitled to one or more debentures under this Act, pursuant to the regulations and restrictions herein before mentioned, and all such sums of their proper money as they shall have actually expended in carrying on or completing such works respectively."

works within said 18 months, and proving the same as herein, to be allowed the same in their deposite;

after six months from 24 June 1789 to be entitled to debentures pursuant to regulations before recited.

" PROVIDED always, and be it further enacted, that no such bodies corporate shall be entitled to any benefits under this Act, save as aforesaid, who shall not have deposited with the Governor and Company of the Bank of Ireland, either in money or by government securities, or shall have actually expended on such works as aforesaid, such tenth part of their respective subscriptions, being the sum for which such bodies corporate respectively are by this act entitled to receive debentures."

Such bodies corporate not entitled to any benefits who have not deposited in the National Bank in money or securities 1-10th of their subscription.

" AND be it further enacted, that if such deposite shall not have been made by such bodies corporate, and if the whole thereof shall not be expended as aforesaid on

If such deposite be not made and the whole expended in 18

months, such part thereof as is not expended to be forfeited to His Majesty.

on such works, within eighteen calendar months after such deposite shall have been so made, that then a moiety of such deposite, or of such part thereof, as shall not have been expended on such works within such time, shall be forfeited to his Majesty, his heirs and successors."

Governor and Co. of the Bank to repay to persons making deposites such part thereof as shall be certified to have been expended on such works.

" AND be it enacted, that the Governor and Company of the said Bank shall, from time to time, repay to the person or persons so making such deposites respectively, so much of the same as shall be certified to the said Governor and Company by the Commissioners of Imprest Accounts, to have been expended on such works respectively, by the person or persons who shall have made such deposites."

No higher toll than 1½d. per mile to be paid for every ton weight of corn, &c. brought by any new Canal or Navigation to Dublin; same toll for water carriage, if partly brought by land carriage and partly by water.

" AND be it further enacted, that no higher toll than one penny half penny per mile be paid on every ton weight of corn, meal, malt, or flour, brought to the City of Dublin, either on any new Canal or Navigation made, improved, or completed under this Act, or if partly by Canal and partly by land carriage, no greater toll shall be charged or paid on the Canal Carriage only."

" AND be it further enacted, that if the charges on the said sum of two hundred thousand pounds sterling, shall not amount to the whole of the said sum, the

propor-

proportions not applied for fhall be granted to fuch future applications, for the
purpofes of Navigation only, as fhall
meet the approbation of Parliament, and
fhall be depofited with the Clerk of the
Houfe of Commons before the firft day of
the meeting of Parliament, in the year
one thoufand feven hundred and ninety-
one."

" AND be it enacted, That fo foon as
any Subfcribers to any of the faid undertakings fhall be conftituted and created
into a body corporate, they fhall be, and
ftand invefted with, and fhall hold and
enjoy all and fingular the like powers,
privileges, advantages, and authorities in
all things, for the purpofes of carrying
on the faid navigations and off-branches,
as were before the paffing of this act
vefted in the corporation for promoting
and carrying on an inland navigation in
Ireland, by virtue of the feveral acts of
parliament heretofore paffed in this kingdom, relative to and concerning inland
navigation, and as are now vefted by
law in the Company of Undertakers of
the Grand Canal, for the purpofe of
enabling them to carry on the faid Canal;
and alfo the like powers as were by the
faid acts heretofore vefted in the faid corporation for promoting and carrying on
an inland navigation in Ireland, and as
are now vefted in the faid Company of
Undertakers

Margin: If the char-ges on the faid fum of 200,000l. fhall not a-mount to the whole of faid fum, fuch part not ap-plied for fhall be difpofed of to fuch appli-cations of a fimilar kind, and fhall be depofited with the clerk of the houfe of commons be-fore the 1ft day of the meeting of parliament in 1791.

When fub-fcribers fhall be conftitut-ed a body corporate, they fhall be vefted with fuch powers as were here-tofore vefted in the corpo-ration for carrying on Inland Na-vigations, and as are now vefted in

Grand Canal Company; with like powers as were vested in corporation for Inland Navigation and Grand Canal Companies to summon juries to value lands, &c.

Undertakers of the Grand Canal, to enable them to summon juries for the valuing any lands, houses, gardens, tenements, and hereditaments (gardens, orchards, yards, lawns, walled deer-parks, and planted avenues excepted) as may be necessary for completing the said works, and for making such wharfs, quays, storehouses, market-houses, locks, basons, and docks, and other conveniencies, as may be judged by such Subscribers and Undertakers when incorporated respectively, proper for the said works, and also all such lands as may be necessary for the making of banks, and towing paths for the aforesaid navigations, and that the said Subscribers and Undertakers when in-

Such subscribers empowered to draw into said Navigation all waters, rivulets, &c. as herein,

making compensation for the same to Proprietor of mills or bleach greens, if such mills or bleach greens were erected before 1st of April, 1789

corporated respectively, may be enabled to hold such lands, houses, tenements, and hereditaments, as they shall so purchase; and further that such Subscribers and Undertakers when incorporated, shall be vested with the like powers, to take, turn, and draw into the said navigations and off-branches the waters of all such rivers, rivulets, lakes, and brooks, as may be necessary for carrying on the aforesaid works, first making compensation as by the said acts directed, to the proprietors of any mills or bleach-greens which may be damaged by the said works, provided such mills or bleach-greens were erected before the first day of April, one thousand seven hundred and eighty-nine."

" AND

" And in order to provide for the pay- Interest for
ment of the interest of the said sum of said deben-
two hundred thousand pounds, or such tures to be
paid as
part thereof as shall be issued by the Vice- herein.
Treasurer or Vice-Treasurers, Paymaster
or Paymasters General, his or their Deputy or Deputies, on debentures to carry
an interest after the rate of four pounds per
centum per annum; Be it enacted, That
for so much of the said sum of two hundred thousand pounds, for which debentures shall be issued, there shall be paid at
the receipt of your Majesty's Exchequer,
by the hands of the Vice-Treasurer or
Vice-Treasurers, Paymaster or Paymasters
General, his or their Deputy or Deputies,
at the end of every six calendar months,
to the person or persons entitled to such
debentures, his, her, or their executors,
administrators or assigns, such interest, not
exceeding the rate of four pounds per
centum per annum, and to commence
respectively from the twenty-fourth of
June next, or from such time subsequent
thereto, at which such debentures shall
be issued, without any fee or charge, and
free from all deductions, defalcations, or
abatements whatsoever, until such time as
they shall be respectively paid their prin-
cipal money at one entire payment."

" And be it further enacted, That every Debentures
such debenture so to be issued, shall be for so to be issued
the precise sum of one hundred pounds, to be for
100l. each,
and

and that the debentures fo to be iffued, fhould be numbered in arithmetical progreffion, where the common excefs or difference is to be one, and that the debentures to be iffued, purfuant to this act, fhall not exceed two thoufand in number, fo that the whole fum to be granted by this act fhall not exceed the fum of two hundred thoufand pounds."

not more than 2000

INDEX.

or complaint against any officer, or relative to any Contract or work to be carried on, for borrowing money, or disposing of any property, or reward of any person, 14.

O.

Oath. Qualifying oath of a Member, 18. Qualifying oath of a proxy, 19. Of a granter of a proxy, 20.

Officers of the Company. Court of Directors to declare their eligibility, 33. Not allowed to enter into any Contracts, or security, *ib.*

P.

Parliament, Act of, relative to Royal Canal, 2—4. Extracts from, 37—46.

Petition of the Company for incorporation, with the recitals therein, 1-4.

Profits. Proprietors of joint stock entitled to, in proportion to their respective interests, 24.

Proxy. Any corporate body, possessed of three shares, may appoint, under seal, a proxy, who may act as one of the Members, 15. No proxy of a body corporate obliged to take any of the oaths, 21. Every change of proxy, to be duly entered, thereby annulling former grant, 17. The granter of a proxy to make affidavit, 19.

R

Rates by the Canal. See *Conveyance.*

Repository for the seal, deeds, maps, &c. with three locks, the keys to be kept by three Members, 34. None of which to be taken away, without receipt being entered in the book, 35.

Royal Canal Company——stiled and named, 7 to continue for ever, 6. Persons constituting such in Charter, 6. Vested with like powers and privileges with those of the Inland Navigation and Grand Canal Companies, 3. Have one common seal, 7. May purchase and sell, sue and be sued, ib. Impowered to carry on and complete a Navigation from Dublin to Tarmonbury, 8. To augment its capital, 9. To borrow on debenture security, 27. May draw into said Navigation and Off-Branches the waters of all rivers, &c. necessary for carrying on their works, first making compensation for mills or bleach-greens, 44.

S.

Shares. See *Stock.*

Stock, Capital, 200,000l —— 66,000l. by Parliament, and 134,000l by subscription, 9. May be augmented any sum not exceeding 300,000l. ib To be divided into shares of 100l. each, 11.

Stock, Joint Proprietors of, may bequeath or assign, but the same not deemed valid unless entry be made thereof in Transfer-Book, 24, 25 May

CPSIA information can be obtained
at www.ICGtesting.com
Printed in the USA
BVOW04s2231170917
495139BV00010B/88/P

9 781170 353660